Blood Sugar Tracker

~weekly set up to track daily readings
~ includes images to color for your enjoyment

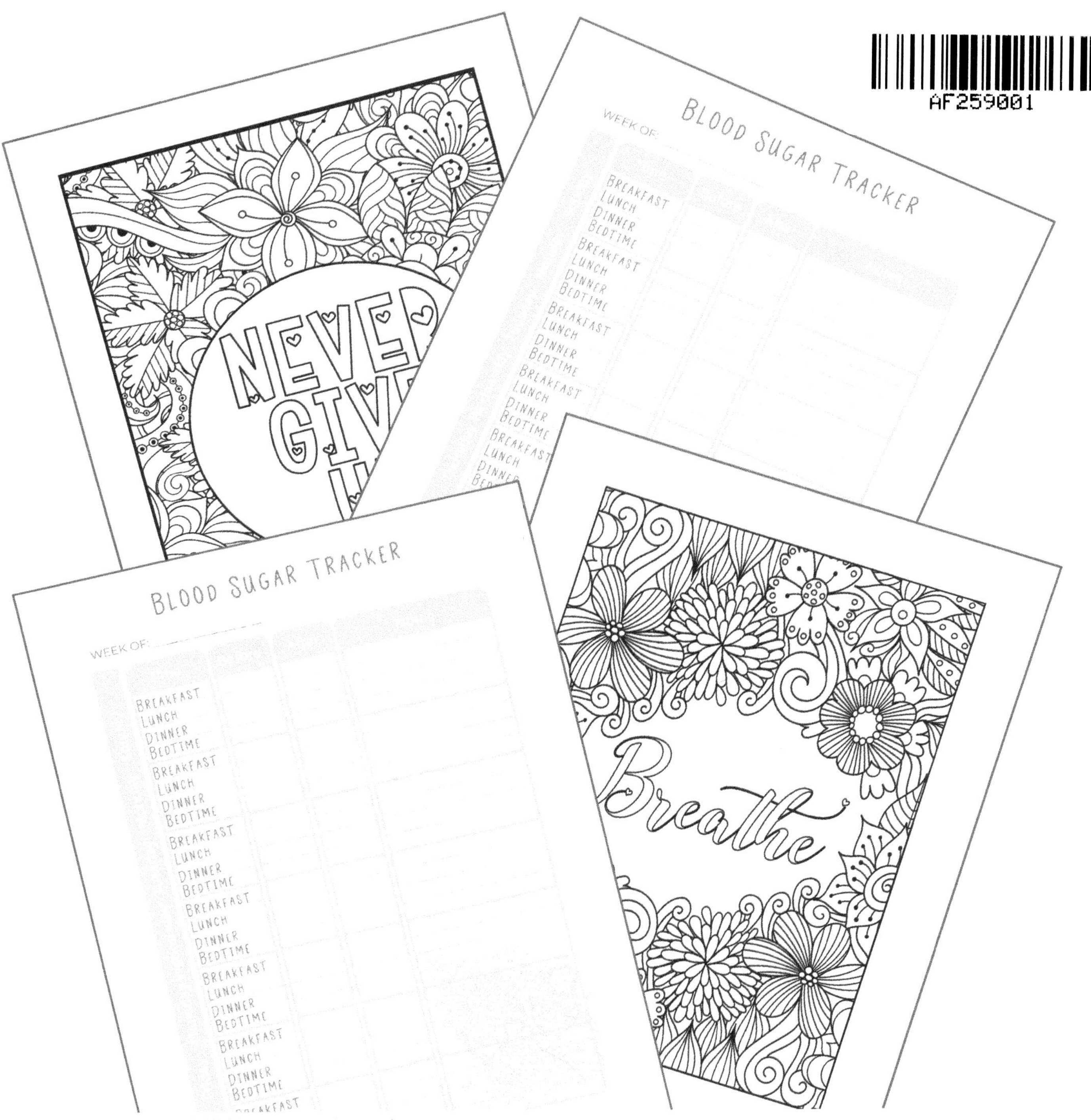

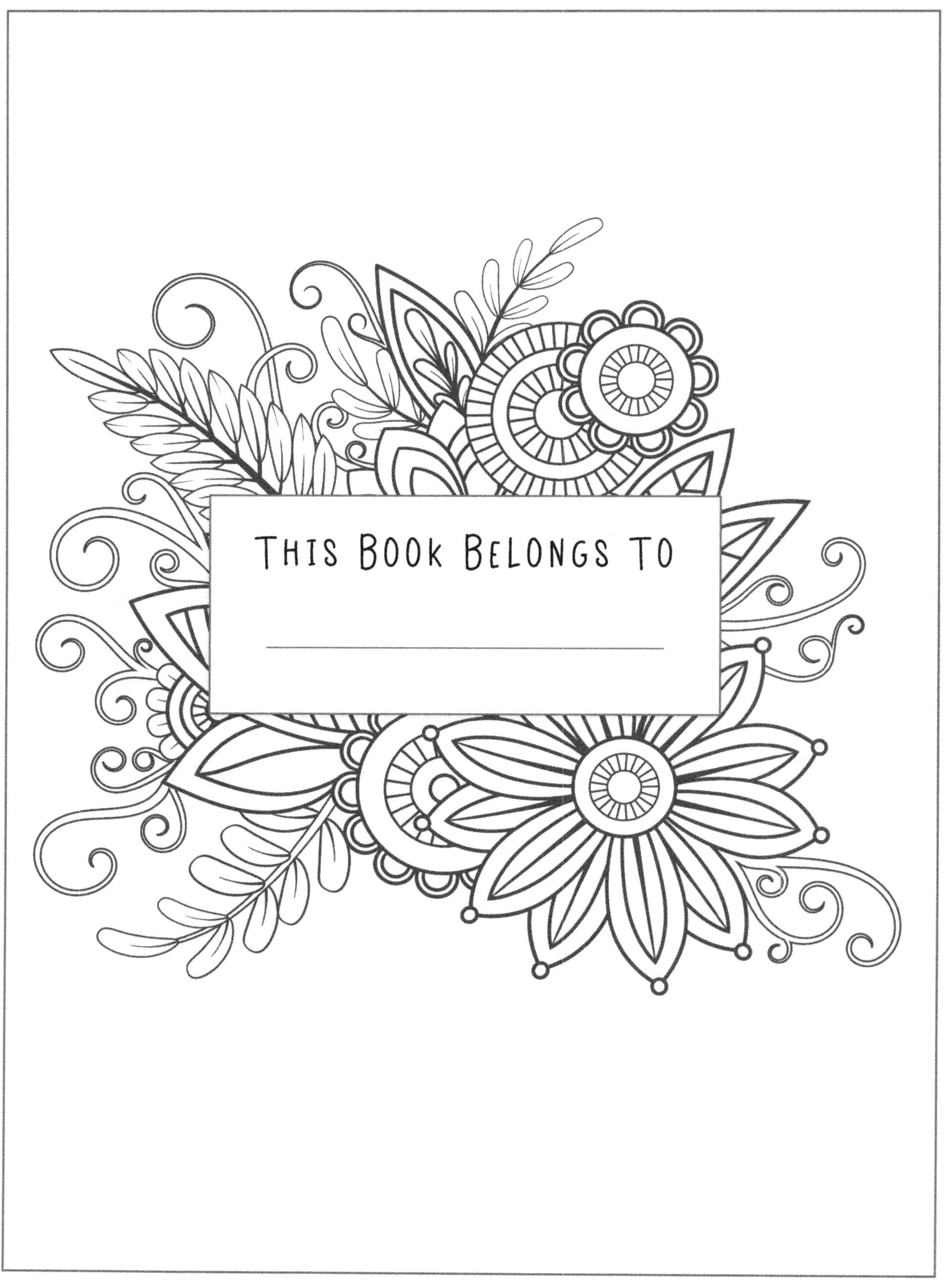
THIS BOOK BELONGS TO

Blood Sugar Tracker

WEEK OF: _________________

	Time	Before	After	Notes
Sunday	Breakfast			
	Lunch			
	Dinner			
	Bedtime			
Monday	Breakfast			
	Lunch			
	Dinner			
	Bedtime			
Tuesday	Breakfast			
	Lunch			
	Dinner			
	Bedtime			
Wednesday	Breakfast			
	Lunch			
	Dinner			
	Bedtime			
Thursday	Breakfast			
	Lunch			
	Dinner			
	Bedtime			
Friday	Breakfast			
	Lunch			
	Dinner			
	Bedtime			
Saturday	Breakfast			
	Lunch			
	Dinner			
	Bedtime			

Blood Sugar Tracker

WEEK OF: _____________________

	Time	Before	After	Notes
Sunday	Breakfast			
	Lunch			
	Dinner			
	Bedtime			
Monday	Breakfast			
	Lunch			
	Dinner			
	Bedtime			
Tuesday	Breakfast			
	Lunch			
	Dinner			
	Bedtime			
Wednesday	Breakfast			
	Lunch			
	Dinner			
	Bedtime			
Thursday	Breakfast			
	Lunch			
	Dinner			
	Bedtime			
Friday	Breakfast			
	Lunch			
	Dinner			
	Bedtime			
Saturday	Breakfast			
	Lunch			
	Dinner			
	Bedtime			

Blood Sugar Tracker

WEEK OF: _________________

	Time	Before	After	Notes
Sunday	Breakfast			
	Lunch			
	Dinner			
	Bedtime			
Monday	Breakfast			
	Lunch			
	Dinner			
	Bedtime			
Tuesday	Breakfast			
	Lunch			
	Dinner			
	Bedtime			
Wednesday	Breakfast			
	Lunch			
	Dinner			
	Bedtime			
Thursday	Breakfast			
	Lunch			
	Dinner			
	Bedtime			
Friday	Breakfast			
	Lunch			
	Dinner			
	Bedtime			
Saturday	Breakfast			
	Lunch			
	Dinner			
	Bedtime			

Blood Sugar Tracker

WEEK OF: _______________________

	Time	Before	After	Notes
Sunday	Breakfast			
	Lunch			
	Dinner			
	Bedtime			
Monday	Breakfast			
	Lunch			
	Dinner			
	Bedtime			
Tuesday	Breakfast			
	Lunch			
	Dinner			
	Bedtime			
Wednesday	Breakfast			
	Lunch			
	Dinner			
	Bedtime			
Thursday	Breakfast			
	Lunch			
	Dinner			
	Bedtime			
Friday	Breakfast			
	Lunch			
	Dinner			
	Bedtime			
Saturday	Breakfast			
	Lunch			
	Dinner			
	Bedtime			

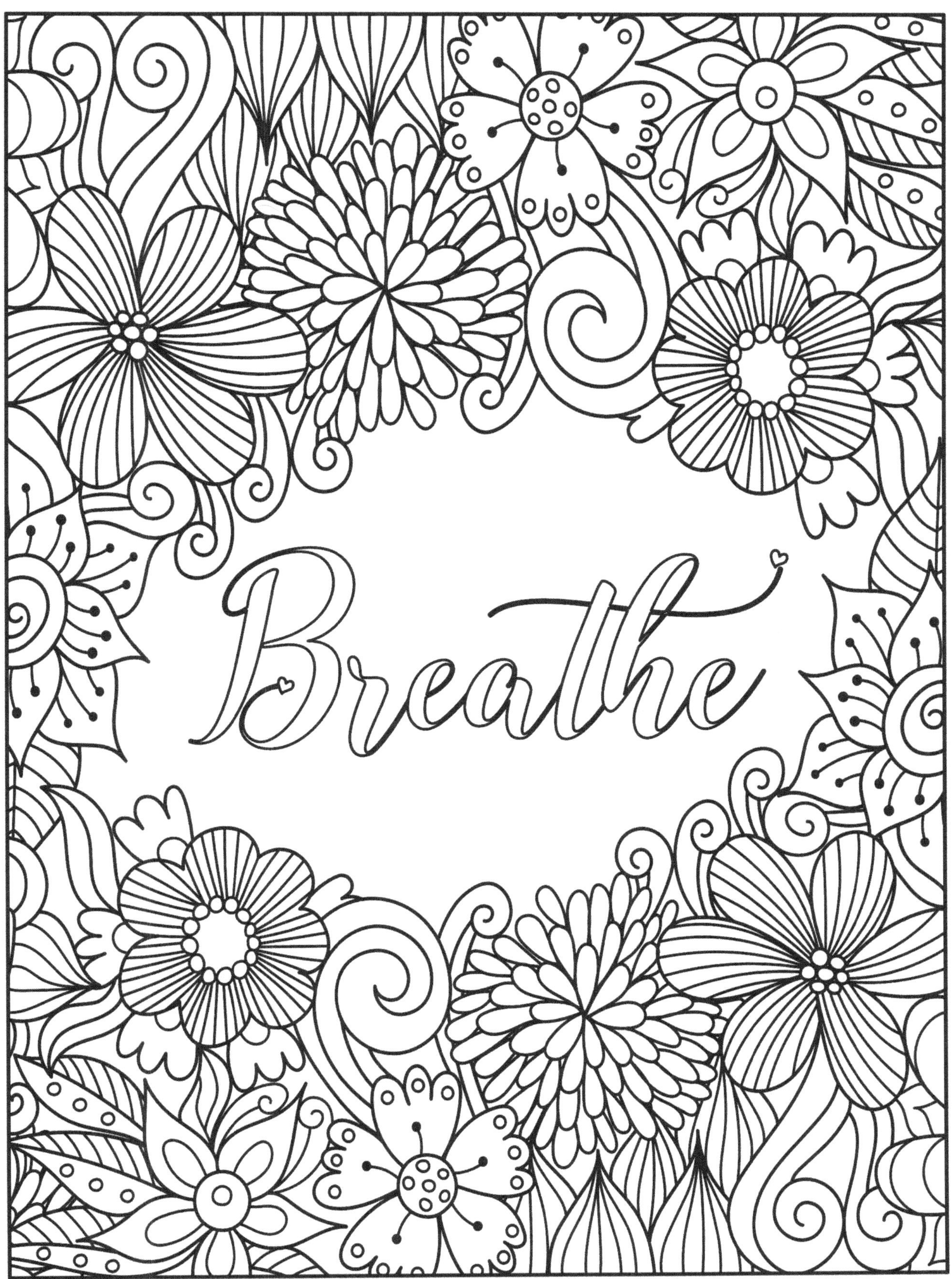
Breathe

Blood Sugar Tracker

WEEK OF: _________________

Time	Before	After	Notes
Breakfast			
Lunch			
Dinner			
Bedtime			
Breakfast			
Lunch			
Dinner			
Bedtime			
Breakfast			
Lunch			
Dinner			
Bedtime			
Breakfast			
Lunch			
Dinner			
Bedtime			
Breakfast			
Lunch			
Dinner			
Bedtime			
Breakfast			
Lunch			
Dinner			
Bedtime			
Breakfast			
Lunch			
Dinner			
Bedtime			

Blood Sugar Tracker

WEEK OF: _______________________

	Time	Before	After	Notes
Sunday	Breakfast Lunch Dinner Bedtime			
Monday	Breakfast Lunch Dinner Bedtime			
Tuesday	Breakfast Lunch Dinner Bedtime			
Wednesday	Breakfast Lunch Dinner Bedtime			
Thursday	Breakfast Lunch Dinner Bedtime			
Friday	Breakfast Lunch Dinner Bedtime			
Saturday	Breakfast Lunch Dinner Bedtime			

Blood Sugar Tracker

WEEK OF: _______________________

	Time	Before	After	Notes
	Breakfast			
	Lunch			
	Dinner			
	Bedtime			
	Breakfast			
	Lunch			
	Dinner			
	Bedtime			
	Breakfast			
	Lunch			
	Dinner			
	Bedtime			
	Breakfast			
	Lunch			
	Dinner			
	Bedtime			
	Breakfast			
	Lunch			
	Dinner			
	Bedtime			
	Breakfast			
	Lunch			
	Dinner			
	Bedtime			
	Breakfast			
	Lunch			
	Dinner			
	Bedtime			

Blood Sugar Tracker

WEEK OF: _________________

	Time	Before	After	Notes
Sunday	Breakfast			
	Lunch			
	Dinner			
	Bedtime			
Monday	Breakfast			
	Lunch			
	Dinner			
	Bedtime			
Tuesday	Breakfast			
	Lunch			
	Dinner			
	Bedtime			
Wednesday	Breakfast			
	Lunch			
	Dinner			
	Bedtime			
Thursday	Breakfast			
	Lunch			
	Dinner			
	Bedtime			
Friday	Breakfast			
	Lunch			
	Dinner			
	Bedtime			
Saturday	Breakfast			
	Lunch			
	Dinner			
	Bedtime			

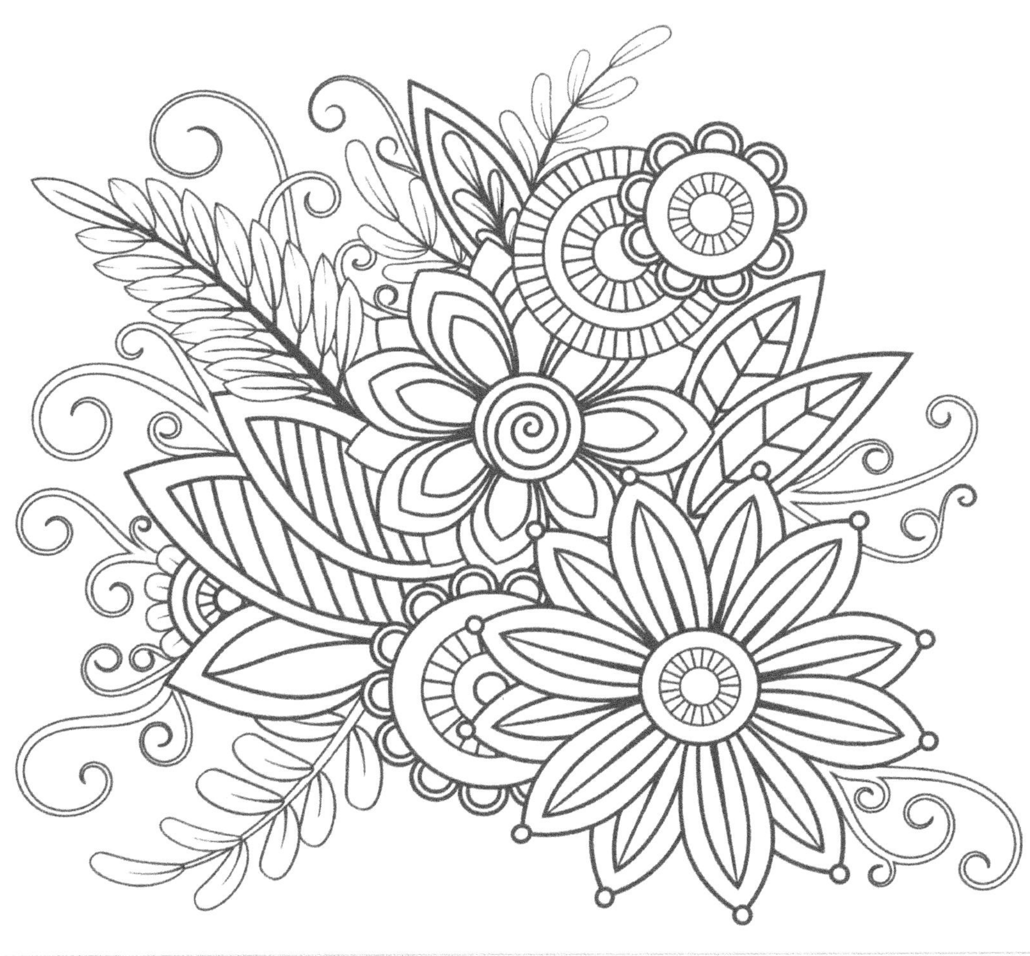

NOTES:

Blood Sugar Tracker

WEEK OF: ______________________

	Time	Before	After	Notes
Sunday	Breakfast Lunch Dinner Bedtime			
Monday	Breakfast Lunch Dinner Bedtime			
Tuesday	Breakfast Lunch Dinner Bedtime			
Wednesday	Breakfast Lunch Dinner Bedtime			
Thursday	Breakfast Lunch Dinner Bedtime			
Friday	Breakfast Lunch Dinner Bedtime			
Saturday	Breakfast Lunch Dinner Bedtime			

Blood Sugar Tracker

WEEK OF: _______________________

	Time	Before	After	Notes
Sunday	Breakfast			
	Lunch			
	Dinner			
	Bedtime			
Monday	Breakfast			
	Lunch			
	Dinner			
	Bedtime			
Tuesday	Breakfast			
	Lunch			
	Dinner			
	Bedtime			
Wednesday	Breakfast			
	Lunch			
	Dinner			
	Bedtime			
Thursday	Breakfast			
	Lunch			
	Dinner			
	Bedtime			
Friday	Breakfast			
	Lunch			
	Dinner			
	Bedtime			
Saturday	Breakfast			
	Lunch			
	Dinner			
	Bedtime			

Blood Sugar Tracker

WEEK OF: _______________________

	Time	Before	After	Notes
SUNDAY	Breakfast Lunch Dinner Bedtime			
MONDAY	Breakfast Lunch Dinner Bedtime			
TUESDAY	Breakfast Lunch Dinner Bedtime			
WEDNESDAY	Breakfast Lunch Dinner Bedtime			
THURSDAY	Breakfast Lunch Dinner Bedtime			
FRIDAY	Breakfast Lunch Dinner Bedtime			
SATURDAY	Breakfast Lunch Dinner Bedtime			

Blood Sugar Tracker

WEEK OF: _______________________

	Time	Before	After	Notes
Sunday	Breakfast			
	Lunch			
	Dinner			
	Bedtime			
Monday	Breakfast			
	Lunch			
	Dinner			
	Bedtime			
Tuesday	Breakfast			
	Lunch			
	Dinner			
	Bedtime			
Wednesday	Breakfast			
	Lunch			
	Dinner			
	Bedtime			
Thursday	Breakfast			
	Lunch			
	Dinner			
	Bedtime			
Friday	Breakfast			
	Lunch			
	Dinner			
	Bedtime			
Saturday	Breakfast			
	Lunch			
	Dinner			
	Bedtime			

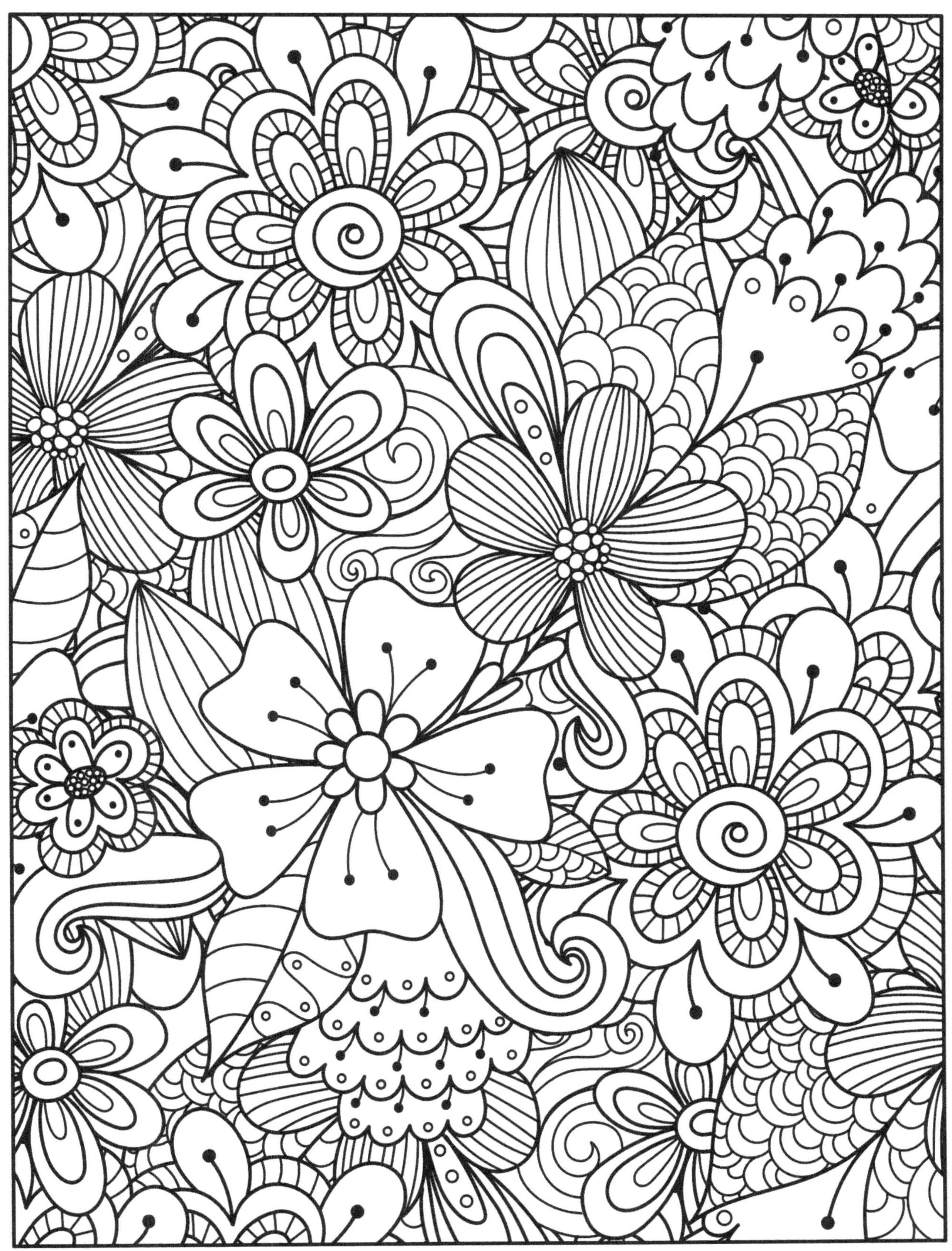

Blood Sugar Tracker

WEEK OF: _______________

	Time	Before	After	Notes
	Breakfast			
	Lunch			
	Dinner			
	Bedtime			
	Breakfast			
	Lunch			
	Dinner			
	Bedtime			
	Breakfast			
	Lunch			
	Dinner			
	Bedtime			
	Breakfast			
	Lunch			
	Dinner			
	Bedtime			
	Breakfast			
	Lunch			
	Dinner			
	Bedtime			
	Breakfast			
	Lunch			
	Dinner			
	Bedtime			
	Breakfast			
	Lunch			
	Dinner			
	Bedtime			

Blood Sugar Tracker

WEEK OF: ___________________

	Time	Before	After	Notes
Sunday	Breakfast			
	Lunch			
	Dinner			
	Bedtime			
Monday	Breakfast			
	Lunch			
	Dinner			
	Bedtime			
Tuesday	Breakfast			
	Lunch			
	Dinner			
	Bedtime			
Wednesday	Breakfast			
	Lunch			
	Dinner			
	Bedtime			
Thursday	Breakfast			
	Lunch			
	Dinner			
	Bedtime			
Friday	Breakfast			
	Lunch			
	Dinner			
	Bedtime			
Saturday	Breakfast			
	Lunch			
	Dinner			
	Bedtime			

Blood Sugar Tracker

WEEK OF: _______________________

BREAKFAST				
LUNCH				
DINNER				
BEDTIME				
BREAKFAST				
LUNCH				
DINNER				
BEDTIME				
BREAKFAST				
LUNCH				
DINNER				
BEDTIME				
BREAKFAST				
LUNCH				
DINNER				
BEDTIME				
BREAKFAST				
LUNCH				
DINNER				
BEDTIME				
BREAKFAST				
LUNCH				
DINNER				
BEDTIME				
BREAKFAST				
LUNCH				
DINNER				
BEDTIME				

Blood Sugar Tracker

WEEK OF: _________________

	Time	Before	After	Notes
Sunday	Breakfast Lunch Dinner Bedtime			
Monday	Breakfast Lunch Dinner Bedtime			
Tuesday	Breakfast Lunch Dinner Bedtime			
Wednesday	Breakfast Lunch Dinner Bedtime			
Thursday	Breakfast Lunch Dinner Bedtime			
Friday	Breakfast Lunch Dinner Bedtime			
Saturday	Breakfast Lunch Dinner Bedtime			

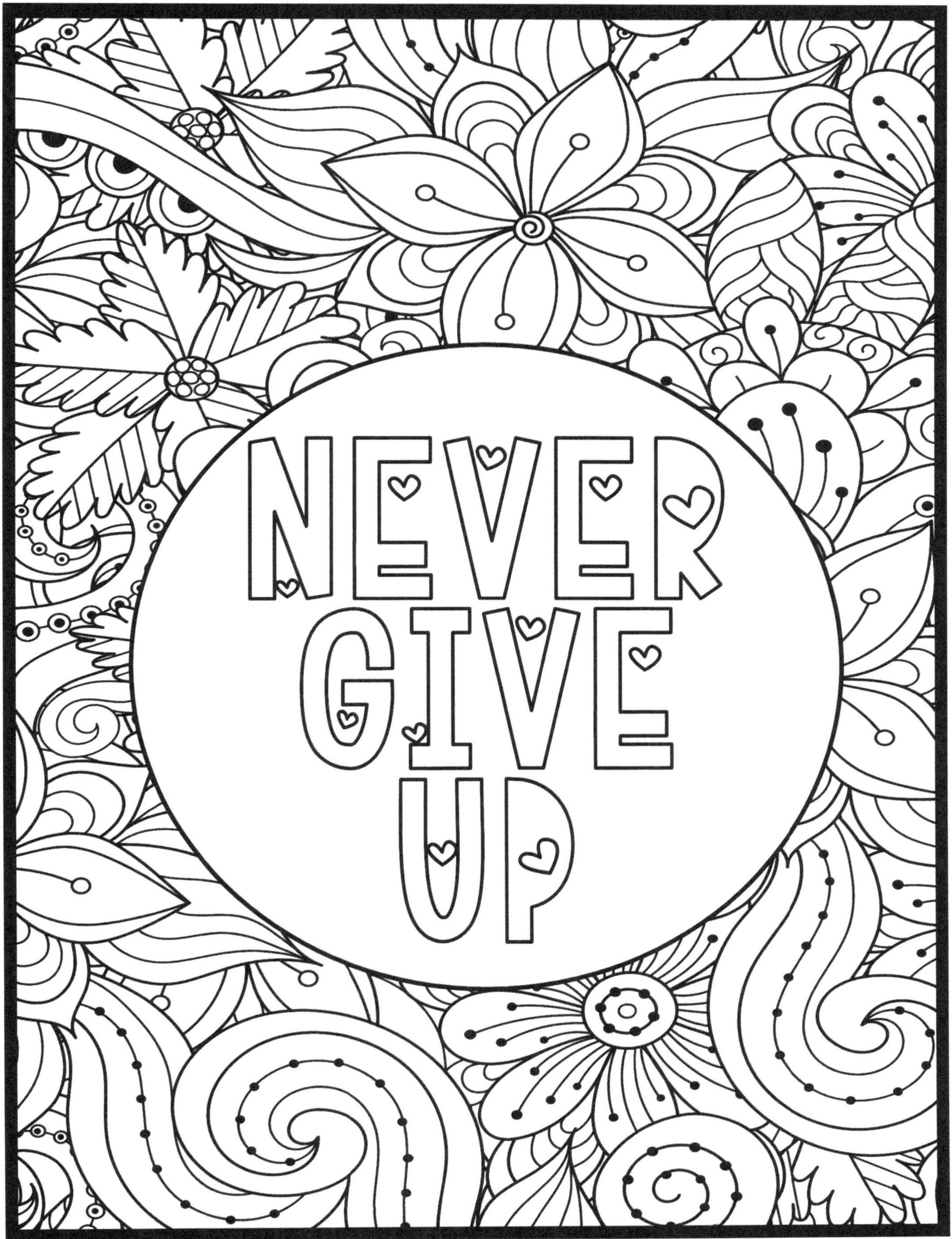

NEVER
GIVE
UP

Blood Sugar Tracker

WEEK OF: _______________

TIME	BEFORE	AFTER	NOTES
Breakfast			
Lunch			
Dinner			
Bedtime			
Breakfast			
Lunch			
Dinner			
Bedtime			
Breakfast			
Lunch			
Dinner			
Bedtime			
Breakfast			
Lunch			
Dinner			
Bedtime			
Breakfast			
Lunch			
Dinner			
Bedtime			
Breakfast			
Lunch			
Dinner			
Bedtime			
Breakfast			
Lunch			
Dinner			
Bedtime			

BLOOD SUGAR TRACKER

WEEK OF: _________________

	Time	Before	After	Notes
Sunday	BREAKFAST LUNCH DINNER BEDTIME			
Monday	BREAKFAST LUNCH DINNER BEDTIME			
Tuesday	BREAKFAST LUNCH DINNER BEDTIME			
Wednesday	BREAKFAST LUNCH DINNER BEDTIME			
Thursday	BREAKFAST LUNCH DINNER BEDTIME			
Friday	BREAKFAST LUNCH DINNER BEDTIME			
Saturday	BREAKFAST LUNCH DINNER BEDTIME			

Blood Sugar Tracker

WEEK OF: _______________

	Time	Before	After	Notes
Sunday	Breakfast			
	Lunch			
	Dinner			
	Bedtime			
Monday	Breakfast			
	Lunch			
	Dinner			
	Bedtime			
Tuesday	Breakfast			
	Lunch			
	Dinner			
	Bedtime			
Wednesday	Breakfast			
	Lunch			
	Dinner			
	Bedtime			
Thursday	Breakfast			
	Lunch			
	Dinner			
	Bedtime			
Friday	Breakfast			
	Lunch			
	Dinner			
	Bedtime			
Saturday	Breakfast			
	Lunch			
	Dinner			
	Bedtime			

Blood Sugar Tracker

WEEK OF: _________________________

Time	Before	After	Notes
Breakfast			
Lunch			
Dinner			
Bedtime			
Breakfast			
Lunch			
Dinner			
Bedtime			
Breakfast			
Lunch			
Dinner			
Bedtime			
Breakfast			
Lunch			
Dinner			
Bedtime			
Breakfast			
Lunch			
Dinner			
Bedtime			
Breakfast			
Lunch			
Dinner			
Bedtime			
Breakfast			
Lunch			
Dinner			
Bedtime			

NOTES:

Blood Sugar Tracker

WEEK OF: _________________________

	Time	Before	After	Notes
Sunday	Breakfast			
	Lunch			
	Dinner			
	Bedtime			
Monday	Breakfast			
	Lunch			
	Dinner			
	Bedtime			
Tuesday	Breakfast			
	Lunch			
	Dinner			
	Bedtime			
Wednesday	Breakfast			
	Lunch			
	Dinner			
	Bedtime			
Thursday	Breakfast			
	Lunch			
	Dinner			
	Bedtime			
Friday	Breakfast			
	Lunch			
	Dinner			
	Bedtime			
Saturday	Breakfast			
	Lunch			
	Dinner			
	Bedtime			

Blood Sugar Tracker

WEEK OF: _______________________

	Time	Before	After	Notes
Sunday	Breakfast Lunch Dinner Bedtime			
Monday	Breakfast Lunch Dinner Bedtime			
Tuesday	Breakfast Lunch Dinner Bedtime			
Wednesday	Breakfast Lunch Dinner Bedtime			
Thursday	Breakfast Lunch Dinner Bedtime			
Friday	Breakfast Lunch Dinner Bedtime			
Saturday	Breakfast Lunch Dinner Bedtime			

Blood Sugar Tracker

WEEK OF: _______________________

	Eating	Before	After	Notes
Sunday	Breakfast			
	Lunch			
	Dinner			
	Bedtime			
Monday	Breakfast			
	Lunch			
	Dinner			
	Bedtime			
Tuesday	Breakfast			
	Lunch			
	Dinner			
	Bedtime			
Wednesday	Breakfast			
	Lunch			
	Dinner			
	Bedtime			
Thursday	Breakfast			
	Lunch			
	Dinner			
	Bedtime			
Friday	Breakfast			
	Lunch			
	Dinner			
	Bedtime			
Saturday	Breakfast			
	Lunch			
	Dinner			
	Bedtime			

Blood Sugar Tracker

WEEK OF: _______________________

	Time	Before	After	Notes
Sunday	Breakfast			
	Lunch			
	Dinner			
	Bedtime			
Monday	Breakfast			
	Lunch			
	Dinner			
	Bedtime			
Tuesday	Breakfast			
	Lunch			
	Dinner			
	Bedtime			
Wednesday	Breakfast			
	Lunch			
	Dinner			
	Bedtime			
Thursday	Breakfast			
	Lunch			
	Dinner			
	Bedtime			
Friday	Breakfast			
	Lunch			
	Dinner			
	Bedtime			
Saturday	Breakfast			
	Lunch			
	Dinner			
	Bedtime			

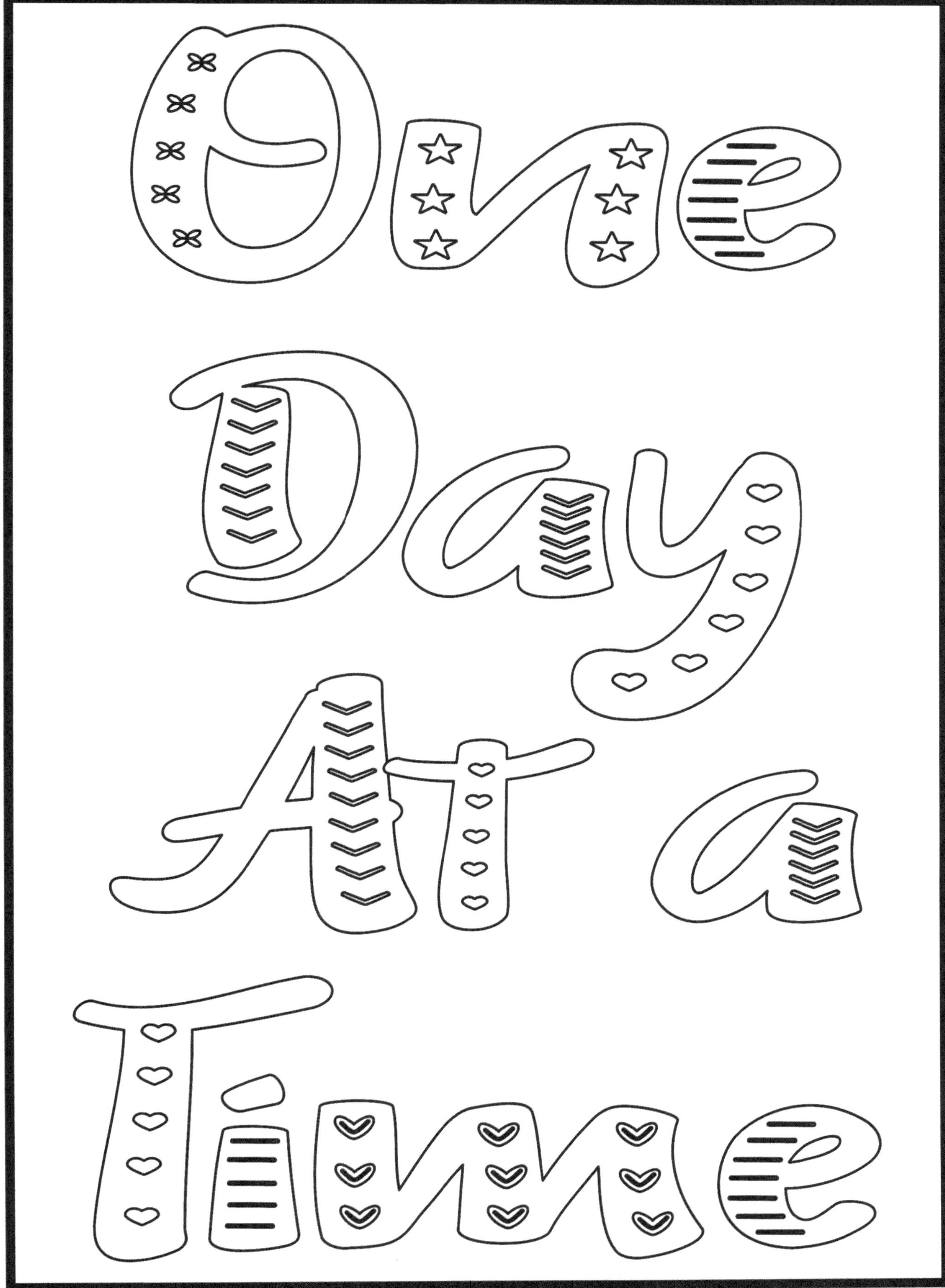

One
Day
At a
Time

Blood Sugar Tracker

WEEK OF: ______________________

	Before	After	Notes
Breakfast			
Lunch			
Dinner			
Bedtime			
Breakfast			
Lunch			
Dinner			
Bedtime			
Breakfast			
Lunch			
Dinner			
Bedtime			
Breakfast			
Lunch			
Dinner			
Bedtime			
Breakfast			
Lunch			
Dinner			
Bedtime			
Breakfast			
Lunch			
Dinner			
Bedtime			
Breakfast			
Lunch			
Dinner			
Bedtime			

Blood Sugar Tracker

WEEK OF: ______________________

	Time	Before	After	Notes
Sunday	BREAKFAST			
	LUNCH			
	DINNER			
	BEDTIME			
Monday	BREAKFAST			
	LUNCH			
	DINNER			
	BEDTIME			
Tuesday	BREAKFAST			
	LUNCH			
	DINNER			
	BEDTIME			
Wednesday	BREAKFAST			
	LUNCH			
	DINNER			
	BEDTIME			
Thursday	BREAKFAST			
	LUNCH			
	DINNER			
	BEDTIME			
Friday	BREAKFAST			
	LUNCH			
	DINNER			
	BEDTIME			
Saturday	BREAKFAST			
	LUNCH			
	DINNER			
	BEDTIME			

Blood Sugar Tracker

WEEK OF: _______________________

	Time	Before	After	Notes
Sunday	Breakfast			
	Lunch			
	Dinner			
	Bedtime			
Monday	Breakfast			
	Lunch			
	Dinner			
	Bedtime			
Tuesday	Breakfast			
	Lunch			
	Dinner			
	Bedtime			
Wednesday	Breakfast			
	Lunch			
	Dinner			
	Bedtime			
Thursday	Breakfast			
	Lunch			
	Dinner			
	Bedtime			
Friday	Breakfast			
	Lunch			
	Dinner			
	Bedtime			
Saturday	Breakfast			
	Lunch			
	Dinner			
	Bedtime			

BLOOD SUGAR TRACKER

WEEK OF: _______________________

	Time	Before	After	Notes
Sunday	BREAKFAST			
	LUNCH			
	DINNER			
	BEDTIME			
Monday	BREAKFAST			
	LUNCH			
	DINNER			
	BEDTIME			
Tuesday	BREAKFAST			
	LUNCH			
	DINNER			
	BEDTIME			
Wednesday	BREAKFAST			
	LUNCH			
	DINNER			
	BEDTIME			
Thursday	BREAKFAST			
	LUNCH			
	DINNER			
	BEDTIME			
Friday	BREAKFAST			
	LUNCH			
	DINNER			
	BEDTIME			
Saturday	BREAKFAST			
	LUNCH			
	DINNER			
	BEDTIME			

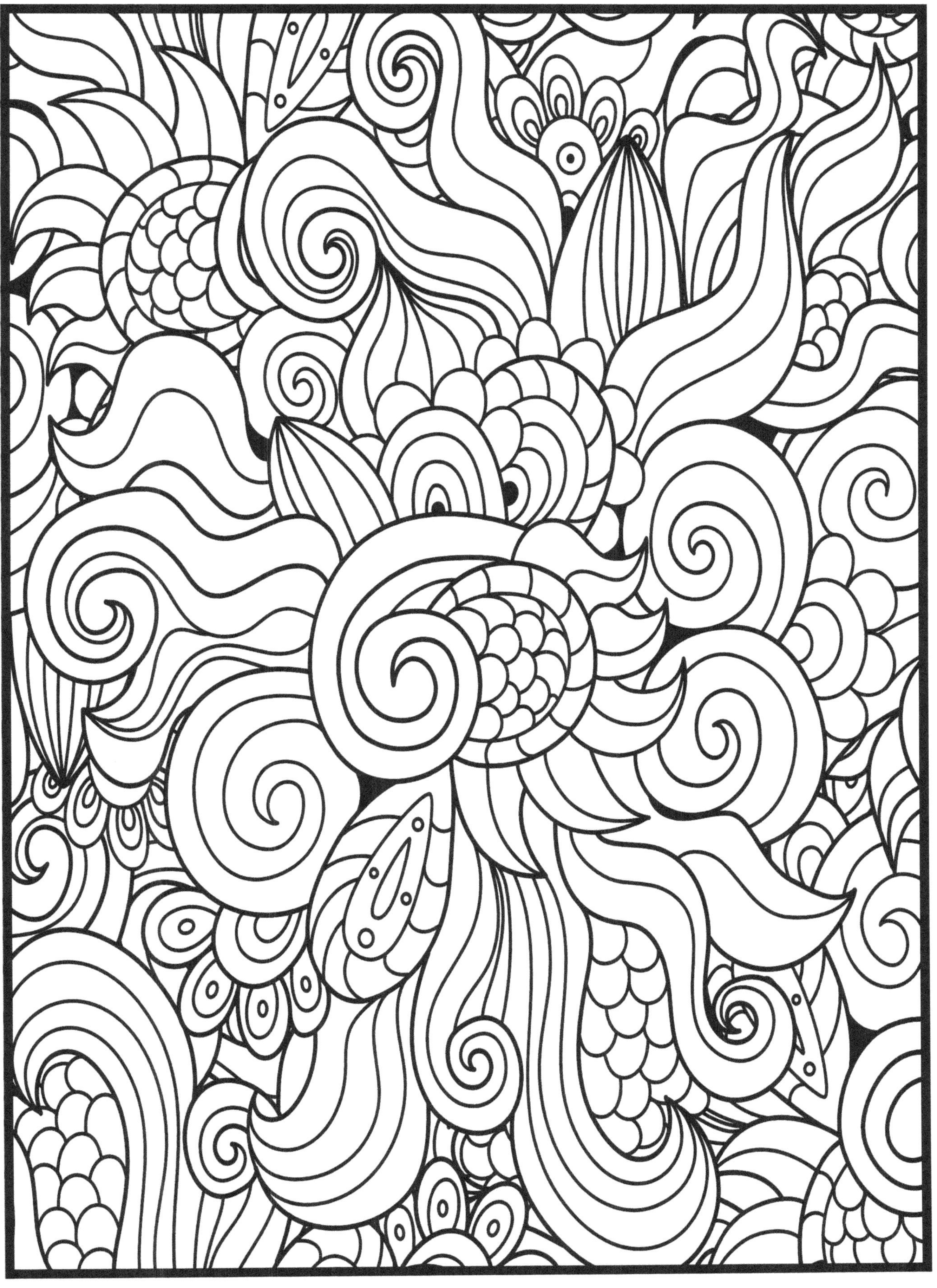

Blood Sugar Tracker

WEEK OF: _____________________

	Time	Before	After	Notes
Sunday	Breakfast Lunch Dinner Bedtime			
Monday	Breakfast Lunch Dinner Bedtime			
Tuesday	Breakfast Lunch Dinner Bedtime			
Wednesday	Breakfast Lunch Dinner Bedtime			
Thursday	Breakfast Lunch Dinner Bedtime			
Friday	Breakfast Lunch Dinner Bedtime			
Saturday	Breakfast Lunch Dinner Bedtime			

Blood Sugar Tracker

WEEK OF: _______________________

Sunday	Time	Before	After	Notes
	Breakfast			
	Lunch			
	Dinner			
	Bedtime			

Monday	Time	Before	After	Notes
	Breakfast			
	Lunch			
	Dinner			
	Bedtime			

Tuesday	Time	Before	After	Notes
	Breakfast			
	Lunch			
	Dinner			
	Bedtime			

Wednesday	Time	Before	After	Notes
	Breakfast			
	Lunch			
	Dinner			
	Bedtime			

Thursday	Time	Before	After	Notes
	Breakfast			
	Lunch			
	Dinner			
	Bedtime			

Friday	Time	Before	After	Notes
	Breakfast			
	Lunch			
	Dinner			
	Bedtime			

Saturday	Time	Before	After	Notes
	Breakfast			
	Lunch			
	Dinner			
	Bedtime			

Blood Sugar Tracker

WEEK OF: ___________________

Time	Before	After	Notes
Breakfast			
Lunch			
Dinner			
Bedtime			
Breakfast			
Lunch			
Dinner			
Bedtime			
Breakfast			
Lunch			
Dinner			
Bedtime			
Breakfast			
Lunch			
Dinner			
Bedtime			
Breakfast			
Lunch			
Dinner			
Bedtime			
Breakfast			
Lunch			
Dinner			
Bedtime			
Breakfast			
Lunch			
Dinner			
Bedtime			

Blood Sugar Tracker

WEEK OF: _______________________

	Time	Before	After	Notes
Sunday	Breakfast			
	Lunch			
	Dinner			
	Bedtime			
Monday	Breakfast			
	Lunch			
	Dinner			
	Bedtime			
Tuesday	Breakfast			
	Lunch			
	Dinner			
	Bedtime			
Wednesday	Breakfast			
	Lunch			
	Dinner			
	Bedtime			
Thursday	Breakfast			
	Lunch			
	Dinner			
	Bedtime			
Friday	Breakfast			
	Lunch			
	Dinner			
	Bedtime			
Saturday	Breakfast			
	Lunch			
	Dinner			
	Bedtime			

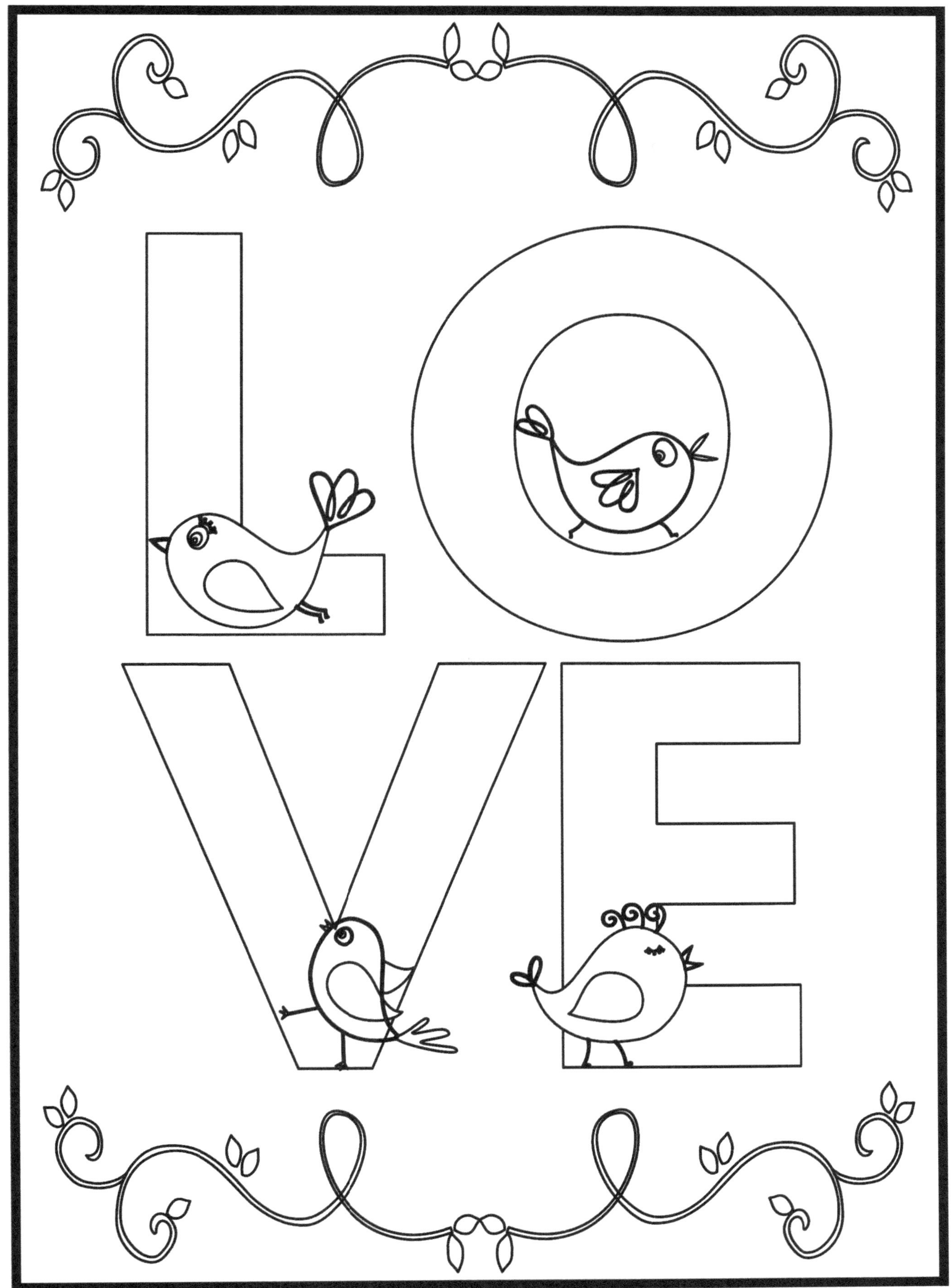

Blood Sugar Tracker

WEEK OF: ___________________

	Time	Before	After	Notes
	Breakfast			
	Lunch			
	Dinner			
	Bedtime			
	Breakfast			
	Lunch			
	Dinner			
	Bedtime			
	Breakfast			
	Lunch			
	Dinner			
	Bedtime			
	Breakfast			
	Lunch			
	Dinner			
	Bedtime			
	Breakfast			
	Lunch			
	Dinner			
	Bedtime			
	Breakfast			
	Lunch			
	Dinner			
	Bedtime			
	Breakfast			
	Lunch			
	Dinner			
	Bedtime			

Blood Sugar Tracker

WEEK OF: _____________________

	Time	Before	After	Notes
Sunday	Breakfast			
	Lunch			
	Dinner			
	Bedtime			
Monday	Breakfast			
	Lunch			
	Dinner			
	Bedtime			
Tuesday	Breakfast			
	Lunch			
	Dinner			
	Bedtime			
Wednesday	Breakfast			
	Lunch			
	Dinner			
	Bedtime			
Thursday	Breakfast			
	Lunch			
	Dinner			
	Bedtime			
Friday	Breakfast			
	Lunch			
	Dinner			
	Bedtime			
Saturday	Breakfast			
	Lunch			
	Dinner			
	Bedtime			

Blood Sugar Tracker

WEEK OF: ________________________

	Time	Before	After	Notes
Sunday	Breakfast			
	Lunch			
	Dinner			
	Bedtime			
Monday	Breakfast			
	Lunch			
	Dinner			
	Bedtime			
Tuesday	Breakfast			
	Lunch			
	Dinner			
	Bedtime			
Wednesday	Breakfast			
	Lunch			
	Dinner			
	Bedtime			
Thursday	Breakfast			
	Lunch			
	Dinner			
	Bedtime			
Friday	Breakfast			
	Lunch			
	Dinner			
	Bedtime			
Saturday	Breakfast			
	Lunch			
	Dinner			
	Bedtime			

Blood Sugar Tracker

WEEK OF: ________________

	Time	Before	After	Notes
Sunday	Breakfast Lunch Dinner Bedtime			
Monday	Breakfast Lunch Dinner Bedtime			
Tuesday	Breakfast Lunch Dinner Bedtime			
Wednesday	Breakfast Lunch Dinner Bedtime			
Thursday	Breakfast Lunch Dinner Bedtime			
Friday	Breakfast Lunch Dinner Bedtime			
Saturday	Breakfast Lunch Dinner Bedtime			

NOTES:

Blood Sugar Tracker

WEEK OF: _________________

	Time	Before	After	Notes
Monday	Breakfast			
	Lunch			
	Dinner			
	Bedtime			
Tuesday	Breakfast			
	Lunch			
	Dinner			
	Bedtime			
Wednesday	Breakfast			
	Lunch			
	Dinner			
	Bedtime			
Thursday	Breakfast			
	Lunch			
	Dinner			
	Bedtime			
Friday	Breakfast			
	Lunch			
	Dinner			
	Bedtime			
Saturday	Breakfast			
	Lunch			
	Dinner			
	Bedtime			
Sunday	Breakfast			
	Lunch			
	Dinner			
	Bedtime			

Blood Sugar Tracker

WEEK OF: _________________________

	Time	Before	After	Notes
Sunday	Breakfast Lunch Dinner Bedtime			
Monday	Breakfast Lunch Dinner Bedtime			
Tuesday	Breakfast Lunch Dinner Bedtime			
Wednesday	Breakfast Lunch Dinner Bedtime			
Thursday	Breakfast Lunch Dinner Bedtime			
Friday	Breakfast Lunch Dinner Bedtime			
Saturday	Breakfast Lunch Dinner Bedtime			

Blood Sugar Tracker

WEEK OF: ________________

Time	Before	After	Notes
Breakfast			
Lunch			
Dinner			
Bedtime			
Breakfast			
Lunch			
Dinner			
Bedtime			
Breakfast			
Lunch			
Dinner			
Bedtime			
Breakfast			
Lunch			
Dinner			
Bedtime			
Breakfast			
Lunch			
Dinner			
Bedtime			
Breakfast			
Lunch			
Dinner			
Bedtime			
Breakfast			
Lunch			
Dinner			
Bedtime			

Blood Sugar Tracker

WEEK OF: _______________________

Time	Before	After	Notes
Breakfast			
Lunch			
Dinner			
Bedtime			
Breakfast			
Lunch			
Dinner			
Bedtime			
Breakfast			
Lunch			
Dinner			
Bedtime			
Breakfast			
Lunch			
Dinner			
Bedtime			
Breakfast			
Lunch			
Dinner			
Bedtime			
Breakfast			
Lunch			
Dinner			
Bedtime			
Breakfast			
Lunch			
Dinner			
Bedtime			

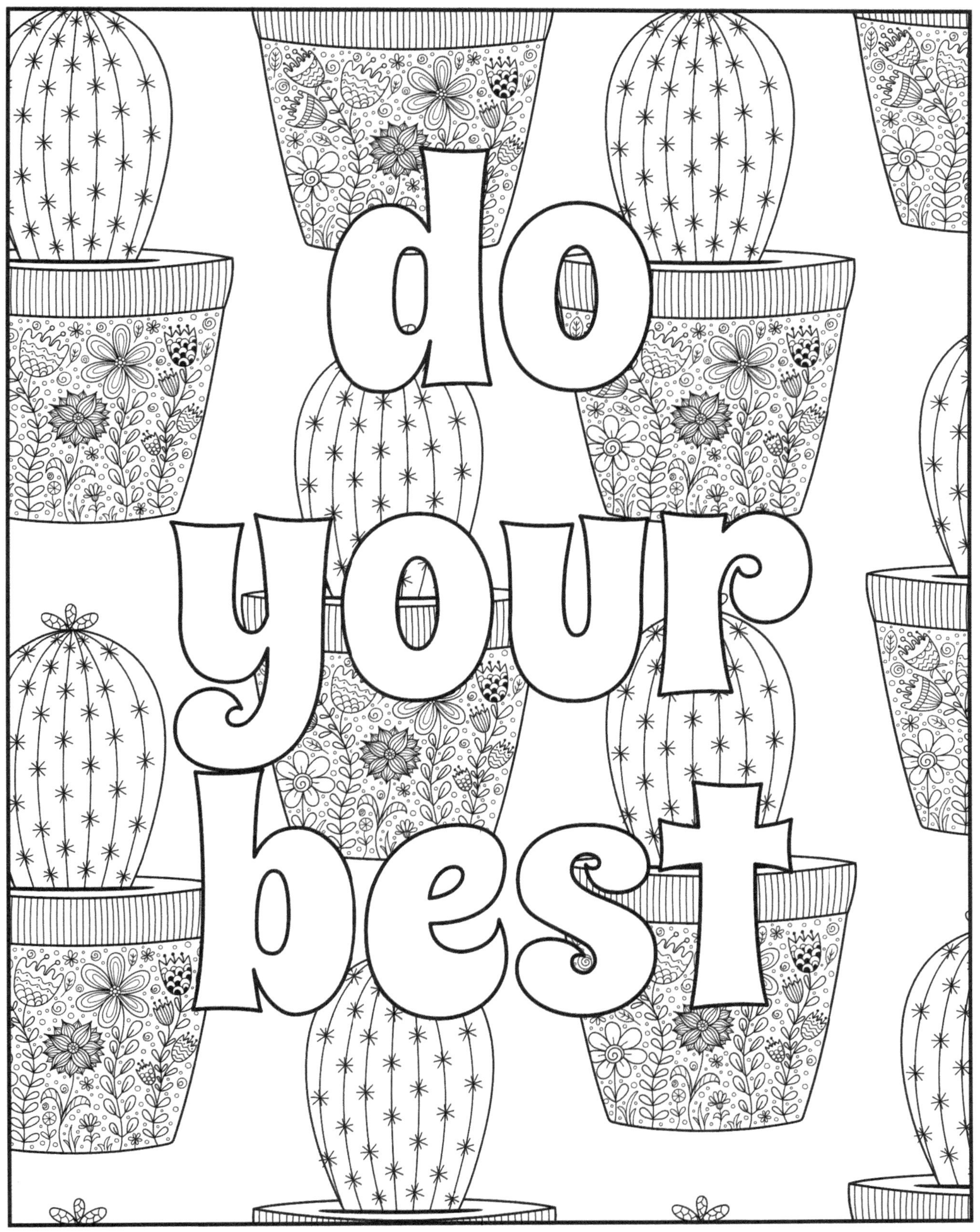

do your best

Blood Sugar Tracker

WEEK OF: _______________________

Time	Before	After	Notes
BREAKFAST			
LUNCH			
DINNER			
BEDTIME			
BREAKFAST			
LUNCH			
DINNER			
BEDTIME			
BREAKFAST			
LUNCH			
DINNER			
BEDTIME			
BREAKFAST			
LUNCH			
DINNER			
BEDTIME			
BREAKFAST			
LUNCH			
DINNER			
BEDTIME			
BREAKFAST			
LUNCH			
DINNER			
BEDTIME			
BREAKFAST			
LUNCH			
DINNER			
BEDTIME			

Blood Sugar Tracker

WEEK OF: _____________________

	Time	Before	After	Notes
Sunday	Breakfast			
	Lunch			
	Dinner			
	Bedtime			
Monday	Breakfast			
	Lunch			
	Dinner			
	Bedtime			
Tuesday	Breakfast			
	Lunch			
	Dinner			
	Bedtime			
Wednesday	Breakfast			
	Lunch			
	Dinner			
	Bedtime			
Thursday	Breakfast			
	Lunch			
	Dinner			
	Bedtime			
Friday	Breakfast			
	Lunch			
	Dinner			
	Bedtime			
Saturday	Breakfast			
	Lunch			
	Dinner			
	Bedtime			

Blood Sugar Tracker

WEEK OF: _______________________

<table>
<tr><td rowspan="28"></td><th>Time</th><th>Before</th><th>After</th><th>Notes</th></tr>
<tr><td>Breakfast</td><td></td><td></td><td></td></tr>
<tr><td>Lunch</td><td></td><td></td><td></td></tr>
<tr><td>Dinner</td><td></td><td></td><td></td></tr>
<tr><td>Bedtime</td><td></td><td></td><td></td></tr>
<tr><td>Breakfast</td><td></td><td></td><td></td></tr>
<tr><td>Lunch</td><td></td><td></td><td></td></tr>
<tr><td>Dinner</td><td></td><td></td><td></td></tr>
<tr><td>Bedtime</td><td></td><td></td><td></td></tr>
<tr><td>Breakfast</td><td></td><td></td><td></td></tr>
<tr><td>Lunch</td><td></td><td></td><td></td></tr>
<tr><td>Dinner</td><td></td><td></td><td></td></tr>
<tr><td>Bedtime</td><td></td><td></td><td></td></tr>
<tr><td>Breakfast</td><td></td><td></td><td></td></tr>
<tr><td>Lunch</td><td></td><td></td><td></td></tr>
<tr><td>Dinner</td><td></td><td></td><td></td></tr>
<tr><td>Bedtime</td><td></td><td></td><td></td></tr>
<tr><td>Breakfast</td><td></td><td></td><td></td></tr>
<tr><td>Lunch</td><td></td><td></td><td></td></tr>
<tr><td>Dinner</td><td></td><td></td><td></td></tr>
<tr><td>Bedtime</td><td></td><td></td><td></td></tr>
<tr><td>Breakfast</td><td></td><td></td><td></td></tr>
<tr><td>Lunch</td><td></td><td></td><td></td></tr>
<tr><td>Dinner</td><td></td><td></td><td></td></tr>
<tr><td>Bedtime</td><td></td><td></td><td></td></tr>
<tr><td>Breakfast</td><td></td><td></td><td></td></tr>
<tr><td>Lunch</td><td></td><td></td><td></td></tr>
<tr><td>Dinner</td><td></td><td></td><td></td></tr>
<tr><td>Bedtime</td><td></td><td></td><td></td></tr>
</table>

Sunday · Monday · Tuesday · Wednesday · Thursday · Friday · Saturday

Blood Sugar Tracker

WEEK OF: _______________________

Time	Before	After	Notes
Breakfast			
Lunch			
Dinner			
Bedtime			
Breakfast			
Lunch			
Dinner			
Bedtime			
Breakfast			
Lunch			
Dinner			
Bedtime			
Breakfast			
Lunch			
Dinner			
Bedtime			
Breakfast			
Lunch			
Dinner			
Bedtime			
Breakfast			
Lunch			
Dinner			
Bedtime			
Breakfast			
Lunch			
Dinner			
Bedtime			

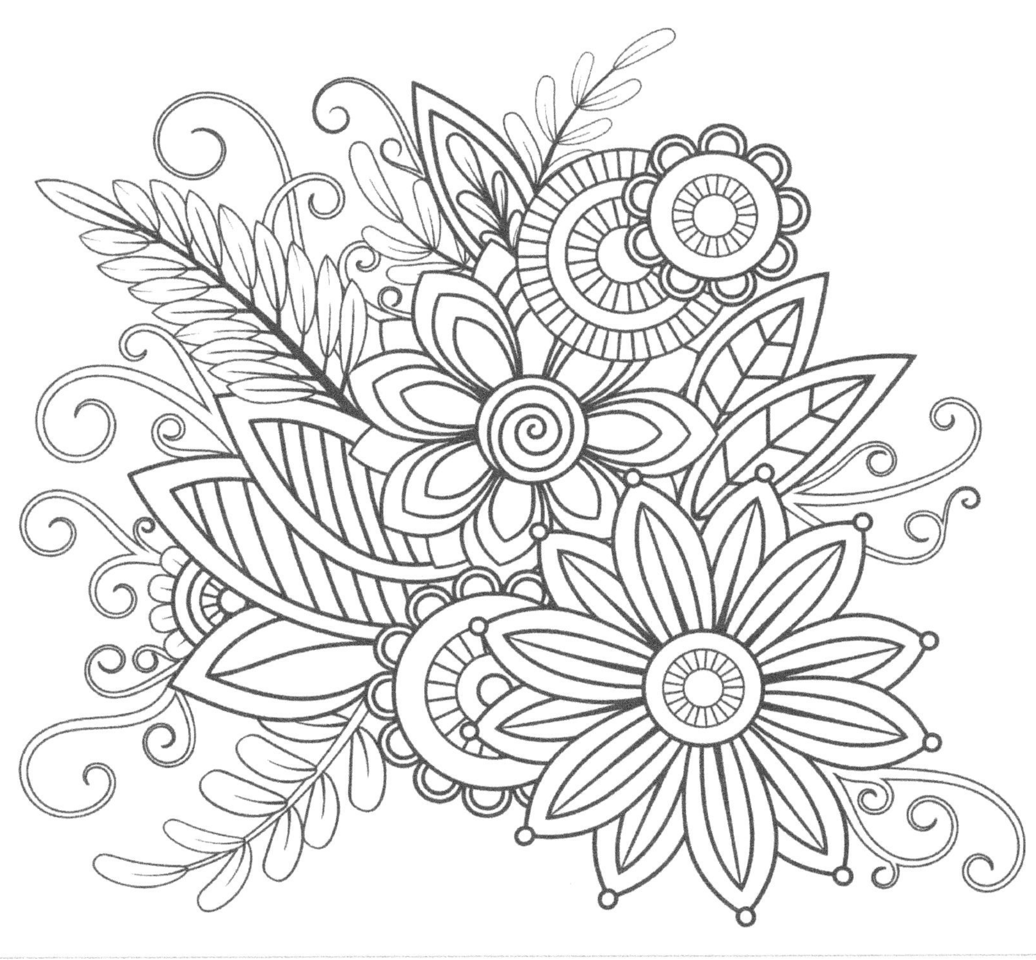

NOTES:

Blood Sugar Tracker

WEEK OF: _______________________

	Time	Before	After	Notes
Sunday	Breakfast Lunch Dinner Bedtime			
Monday	Breakfast Lunch Dinner Bedtime			
Tuesday	Breakfast Lunch Dinner Bedtime			
Wednesday	Breakfast Lunch Dinner Bedtime			
Thursday	Breakfast Lunch Dinner Bedtime			
Friday	Breakfast Lunch Dinner Bedtime			
Saturday	Breakfast Lunch Dinner Bedtime			

Blood Sugar Tracker

WEEK OF: _______________________

	Time	Before	After	Notes
Sunday	Breakfast			
	Lunch			
	Dinner			
	Bedtime			
Monday	Breakfast			
	Lunch			
	Dinner			
	Bedtime			
Tuesday	Breakfast			
	Lunch			
	Dinner			
	Bedtime			
Wednesday	Breakfast			
	Lunch			
	Dinner			
	Bedtime			
Thursday	Breakfast			
	Lunch			
	Dinner			
	Bedtime			
Friday	Breakfast			
	Lunch			
	Dinner			
	Bedtime			
Saturday	Breakfast			
	Lunch			
	Dinner			
	Bedtime			

Blood Sugar Tracker

WEEK OF: _________________________

	Time	Before	After	Notes
Sunday	Breakfast Lunch Dinner Bedtime			
Monday	Breakfast Lunch Dinner Bedtime			
Tuesday	Breakfast Lunch Dinner Bedtime			
Wednesday	Breakfast Lunch Dinner Bedtime			
Thursday	Breakfast Lunch Dinner Bedtime			
Friday	Breakfast Lunch Dinner Bedtime			
Saturday	Breakfast Lunch Dinner Bedtime			

Blood Sugar Tracker

WEEK OF: ________________

	Time	Before	After	Notes
Sunday	Breakfast			
	Lunch			
	Dinner			
	Bedtime			
Monday	Breakfast			
	Lunch			
	Dinner			
	Bedtime			
Tuesday	Breakfast			
	Lunch			
	Dinner			
	Bedtime			
Wednesday	Breakfast			
	Lunch			
	Dinner			
	Bedtime			
Thursday	Breakfast			
	Lunch			
	Dinner			
	Bedtime			
Friday	Breakfast			
	Lunch			
	Dinner			
	Bedtime			
Saturday	Breakfast			
	Lunch			
	Dinner			
	Bedtime			

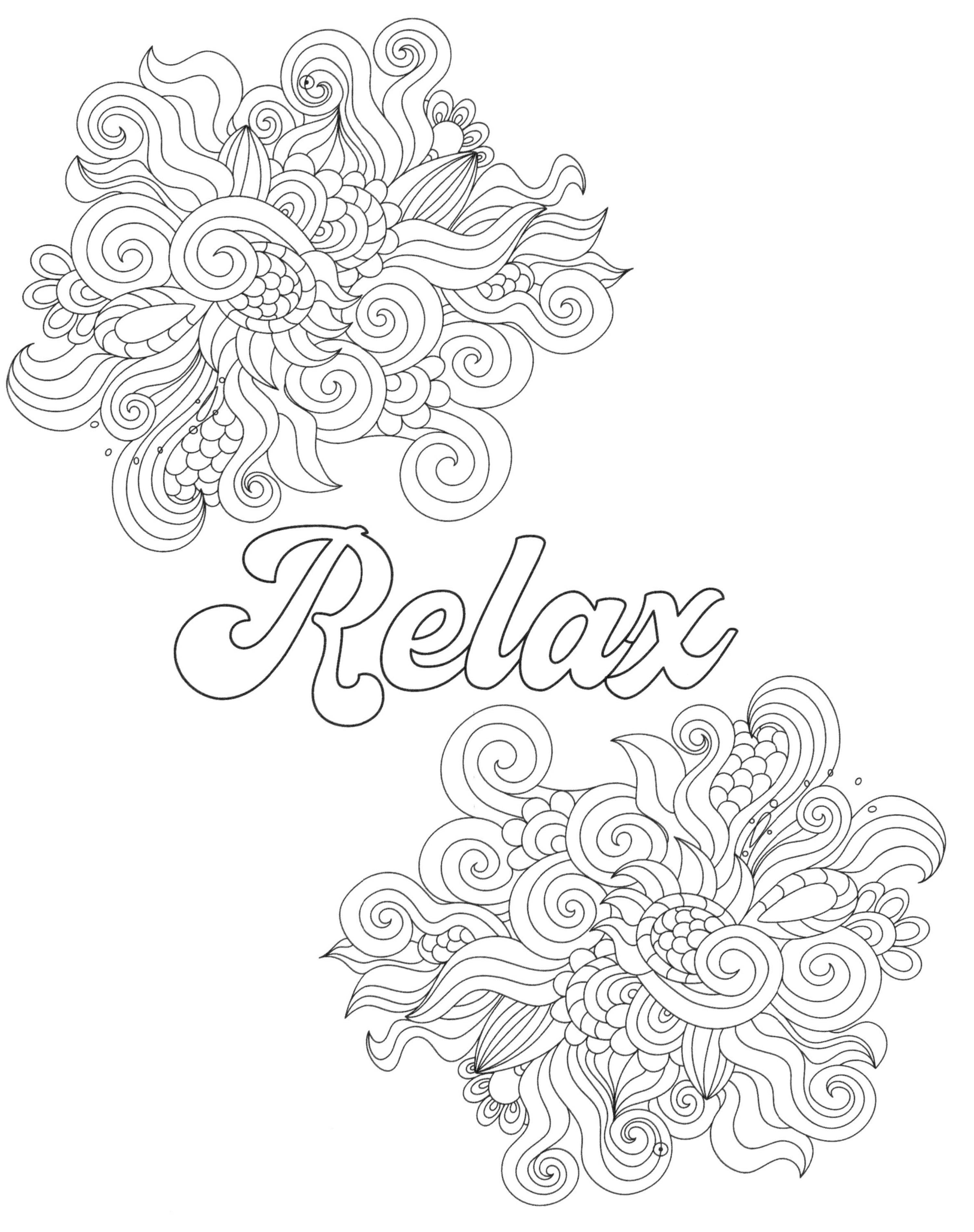
Relax

Blood Sugar Tracker

WEEK OF: ___________________

	Time	Before	After	Notes
	Breakfast			
	Lunch			
	Dinner			
	Bedtime			
	Breakfast			
	Lunch			
	Dinner			
	Bedtime			
	Breakfast			
	Lunch			
	Dinner			
	Bedtime			
	Breakfast			
	Lunch			
	Dinner			
	Bedtime			
	Breakfast			
	Lunch			
	Dinner			
	Bedtime			
	Breakfast			
	Lunch			
	Dinner			
	Bedtime			
	Breakfast			
	Lunch			
	Dinner			
	Bedtime			

Blood Sugar Tracker

WEEK OF: _______________________

	Time	Before	After	Notes
Sunday	Breakfast			
	Lunch			
	Dinner			
	Bedtime			
Monday	Breakfast			
	Lunch			
	Dinner			
	Bedtime			
Tuesday	Breakfast			
	Lunch			
	Dinner			
	Bedtime			
Wednesday	Breakfast			
	Lunch			
	Dinner			
	Bedtime			
Thursday	Breakfast			
	Lunch			
	Dinner			
	Bedtime			
Friday	Breakfast			
	Lunch			
	Dinner			
	Bedtime			
Saturday	Breakfast			
	Lunch			
	Dinner			
	Bedtime			

Blood Sugar Tracker

WEEK OF: _______________________

	Time	Before	After	Notes
Sunday	Breakfast			
	Lunch			
	Dinner			
	Bedtime			
Monday	Breakfast			
	Lunch			
	Dinner			
	Bedtime			
Tuesday	Breakfast			
	Lunch			
	Dinner			
	Bedtime			
Wednesday	Breakfast			
	Lunch			
	Dinner			
	Bedtime			
Thursday	Breakfast			
	Lunch			
	Dinner			
	Bedtime			
Friday	Breakfast			
	Lunch			
	Dinner			
	Bedtime			
Saturday	Breakfast			
	Lunch			
	Dinner			
	Bedtime			

Blood Sugar Tracker

WEEK OF: _______________________

	Time	Before	After	Notes
Sunday	Breakfast Lunch Dinner Bedtime			
Monday	Breakfast Lunch Dinner Bedtime			
Tuesday	Breakfast Lunch Dinner Bedtime			
Wednesday	Breakfast Lunch Dinner Bedtime			
Thursday	Breakfast Lunch Dinner Bedtime			
Friday	Breakfast Lunch Dinner Bedtime			
Saturday	Breakfast Lunch Dinner Bedtime			

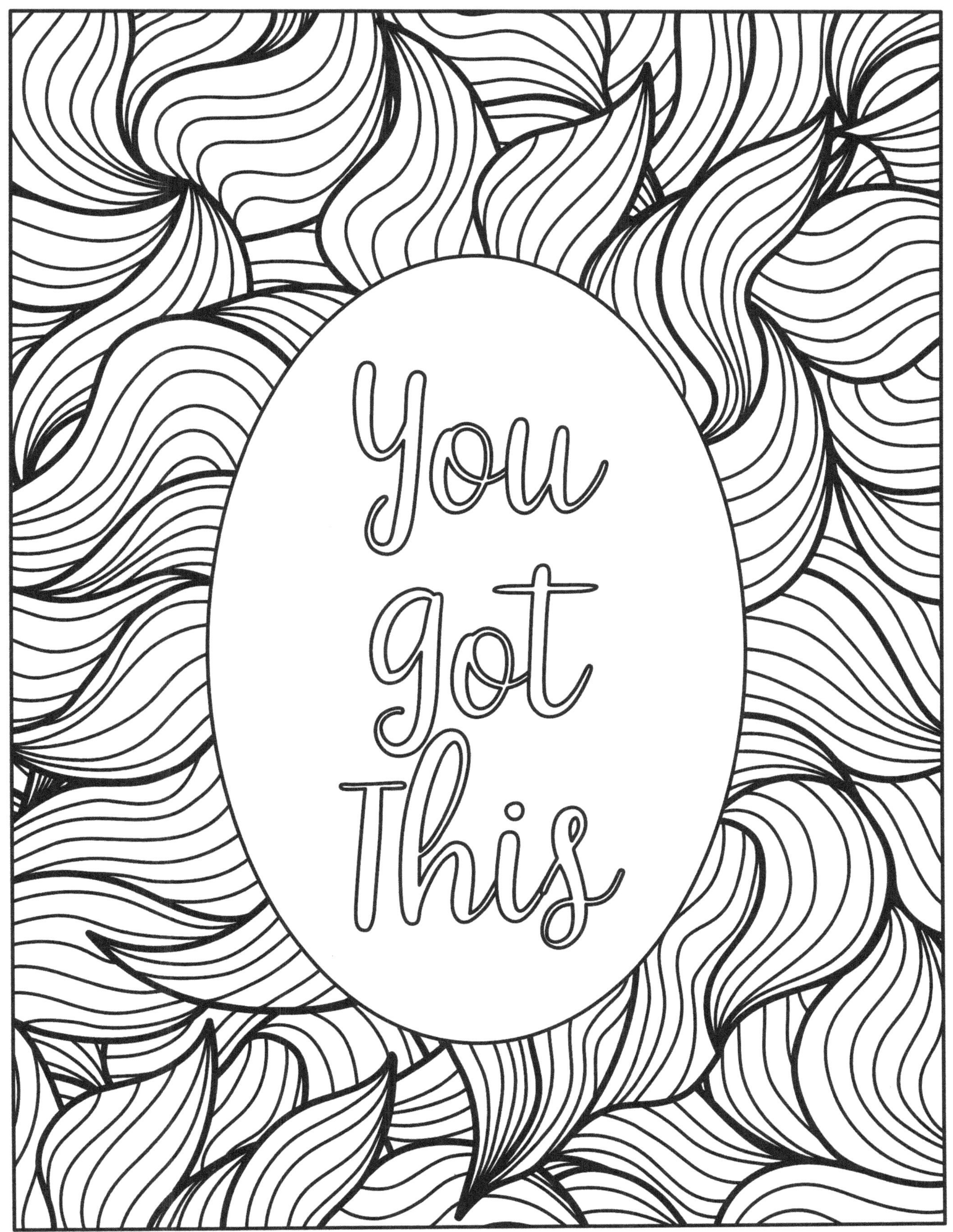

You
got
This

Blood Sugar Tracker

WEEK OF: _______________________

	Time	Before	After	Notes
Sunday	Breakfast Lunch Dinner Bedtime			
Monday	Breakfast Lunch Dinner Bedtime			
Tuesday	Breakfast Lunch Dinner Bedtime			
Wednesday	Breakfast Lunch Dinner Bedtime			
Thursday	Breakfast Lunch Dinner Bedtime			
Friday	Breakfast Lunch Dinner Bedtime			
Saturday	Breakfast Lunch Dinner Bedtime			

BLOOD SUGAR TRACKER

WEEK OF: _______________________

	Time	Before	After	Notes
Sunday	Breakfast			
	Lunch			
	Dinner			
	Bedtime			
Monday	Breakfast			
	Lunch			
	Dinner			
	Bedtime			
Tuesday	Breakfast			
	Lunch			
	Dinner			
	Bedtime			
Wednesday	Breakfast			
	Lunch			
	Dinner			
	Bedtime			
Thursday	Breakfast			
	Lunch			
	Dinner			
	Bedtime			
Friday	Breakfast			
	Lunch			
	Dinner			
	Bedtime			
Saturday	Breakfast			
	Lunch			
	Dinner			
	Bedtime			

Blood Sugar Tracker

WEEK OF: ______________________

Time	Before	After	Notes
Breakfast			
Lunch			
Dinner			
Bedtime			
Breakfast			
Lunch			
Dinner			
Bedtime			
Breakfast			
Lunch			
Dinner			
Bedtime			
Breakfast			
Lunch			
Dinner			
Bedtime			
Breakfast			
Lunch			
Dinner			
Bedtime			
Breakfast			
Lunch			
Dinner			
Bedtime			
Breakfast			
Lunch			
Dinner			
Bedtime			

Blood Sugar Tracker

WEEK OF: ______________________

	Time	Before	After	Notes
Sunday	Breakfast			
	Lunch			
	Dinner			
	Bedtime			
Monday	Breakfast			
	Lunch			
	Dinner			
	Bedtime			
Tuesday	Breakfast			
	Lunch			
	Dinner			
	Bedtime			
Wednesday	Breakfast			
	Lunch			
	Dinner			
	Bedtime			
Thursday	Breakfast			
	Lunch			
	Dinner			
	Bedtime			
Friday	Breakfast			
	Lunch			
	Dinner			
	Bedtime			
Saturday	Breakfast			
	Lunch			
	Dinner			
	Bedtime			

NOTES: